Table of Contents

Hyperthyroidism is a set of disorders that involve excess synthesis and secretion of thyroid hormones by the thyroid gland, which leads to the hypermetabolic condition of thyrotoxicosis. [1, 2] The most common forms of hyperthyroidism include diffuse toxic goiter (Graves disease), toxic multinodular goiter (Plummer disease), and toxic adenoma. In thyrotoxicosis, thyroid hormone levels are elevated with or without increased thyroid hormone synthesis. The most common forms of thyrotoxicosis are caused by excess intake of the thyroid hormone medication levothyroxine or result from a temporary excess release of thyroid hormone due to subacute thyroiditis. The most reliable screening measure of thyroid function is the thyroid-stimulating hormone (TSH) level. Treatment of hyperthyroidism includes symptom relief, as well as antithyroid pharmacotherapy, radioactive iodine-131 (^{131}I) therapy (the preferred treatment of hyperthyroidism among US thyroid specialists), or thyroidectomy. Thyrotoxicosis from subacute thyroiditis is temporary and self-resolving, and the treatment is also symptom relief.

BREAKFAST

1. Collagen Turmeric Chocolate Truffles

Prep Time: 5 Minutes

Cook Time: 20 Minutes

Servings: 12

Ingredients

Tools

- Small paper liners
- Medium mixing bowl
- ½ cup coconut oil, melted
- ½ cup raw cacao powder
- 5 T raw honey
- 2 T collagen powder
- 1 t turmeric powder
- ¼ cup unsweetened shredded coconut

Instructions

1. Melt the coconut oil in a double boiler. Whisk in the cacao powder, raw honey, and collagen powder, mixing well until you get a smooth and shiny chocolate mixture.

2. Chill the mixture in the refrigerator for at least 1 hour until it hardens and the ganache is set (it should be firm, but malleable).

3. While the ganache is chilling, mix the turmeric powder and shredded coconut in a bowl until the shredded coconut is a bright yellow. Set aside.

4. Scoop out 1 tablespoon of the ganache and roll it into a small ball using the palms of your hands. Place the ball onto a plate and set aside. Repeat with the rest of the ganache until it's all used up. If the ganache starts to melt and it becomes hard to roll the balls, chill it in the refrigerator for 5 minutes before rolling again.

5. Roll the balls one by one in the turmeric shredded coconut and coat them all over. Place the truffles into small paper liners and chill for at least 10 minutes before serving.

6. Store the truffles in an airtight container in the refrigerator for up to a week.

Prep Time: 15 Minutes

Cook Time: 30 Minutes

Servings: 8

Ingredients

- 1 Tbsp olive oil
- 3 links raw chicken sausage, casings removed
- 1 small onion, diced
- 2 cloves garlic, minced
- Pinch red pepper flakes
- 1 can (28 oz) crushed tomatoes
- Salt and black pepper to taste
- 1 1/2 cups low-fat ricotta (Barilla makes a good no-boil lasagna that is widely available.)
- 1/2 cup 2% milk
- 16 sheets no-boil lasagna noodles
- 16–20 fresh basil leaves
- 1 cup chopped fresh mozzarella

Instructions

1. Heat the olive oil in a large saucepan over medium heat.

2. Add the sausage and cook for about 3 minutes, until no longer pink.

3. Add the onion, garlic, and red pepper flakes and continue cooking for about 5 minutes, until the onion is soft and translucent.

4. Add the tomatoes and simmer for 15 minutes.

5. Season with salt and pepper.

6. Preheat the oven to 350 degrees Fahrenheit.

7. Combine the ricotta and milk in a mixing bowl.

8. In a 9" x 9" baking pan, lay down a layer of 4 noodles.

9. Cover with a quarter of the ricotta mixture and a quarter of the sausage mixture, then a few basil leaves and a quarter of the mozzarella.

10. Repeat three times to create a four-layer lasagna.

11. Cover with aluminum foil and bake for 25 minutes, until the cheese is melted and the pasta cooked through.

12. Remove the foil and increase the temperature to 450 degrees Fahrenheit.

13. Continue baking for about 10 minutes, until the top of the lasagna is nicely browned.

Prep Time: 15 Minutes

Cook Time: 45 Minutes

Servings: 4

Ingredients

- 3 Tbsp low-sodium soy sauce
- 3 Tbsp oyster sauce
- 2 Tbsp Shaoxing rice wine, sherry, or dry white wine
- 1 Tbsp brown sugar
- 1 tsp toasted sesame oil
- 1 tsp cornstarch
- 1 lb flank steak, thinly sliced
- ½ Tbsp canola or peanut oil
- 1 lb broccoli, broken into bite-size pieces
- 1 red or yellow bell pepper, cored and sliced
- 4 cloves garlic, minced
- 1 Tbsp grated fresh ginger
- ¼ cup low-sodium beef stock

Instructions

1. Combine the soy sauce, oyster sauce, Shaoxing, brown sugar, sesame oil, and cornstarch in a large mixing bowl.

2. Whisk to combine the liquid with the cornstarch.

3. Mix in the beef and let marinate for 30 minutes.

4. Heat the oil in a wok over medium heat.

5. Add the broccoli, bell pepper, garlic, and ginger and stir-fry, using a spatula to keep the vegetables moving, for about 5 minutes, until the vegetables have softened.

6. Add the beef and its marinade and continue cooking, stirring frequently, for about 5 minutes, until the beef is browned and nearly cooked through.

7. Add the stock and cook for another 2 minutes, until the sauce thickens and clings to the beef and vegetables.

8. Serve over steamed brown rice, if you like.

Prep Time: 50 Minutes

Cook Time: 2hrs 50 Minutes

Servings: 6

Ingredients

- 1 19.2-ounce package ground turkey breast
- 1 8-ounce package. cremini mushrooms, coarsely chopped
- 1 28-ounce can no-salt-added diced tomatoes
- 1 15-ounce can kidney beans, rinsed and drained
- 1 15-ounce can black beans, rinsed and drained
- 1 cup chopped onion
- 1 cup chopped green bell pepper
- 1 6-ounce can no-salt-added tomato paste
- 1 tablespoon chili powder
- 2 teaspoon garlic powder
- 1 teaspoon ground cumin
- 1 teaspoon dried oregano, crushed
- 1/2 teaspoon ground chipotle chile pepper
- 1/2 teaspoon salt
- 2 cups chopped zucchini

- Green onions, fresh cilantro, and lime wedges

Instructions

1. In a large nonstick skillet cook turkey and mushrooms over medium until turkey is no longer pink, stirring to break apart. Drain. Place in a 4- to 5-qt. slow cooker. Add tomatoes, both beans, onion, bell pepper, tomato paste, chili powder, garlic powder, cumin, oregano, chipotle chile, and salt. Stir to combine.

2. Cover and cook on low 6 to 8 hours or high 3 to 4 hours. If using low, turn cooker to high, stir in zucchini and cover and cook 30 minutes more or until tender.

3. Top as desired with green onions, cilantro, and lime wedges.

4. nutrition per serving: 298 calories, 2 g fat (0 g saturated fat), 521 mg sodium, 12 g sugar, 12 g fiber, 34 g protein[/nutrinfo-black]

Prep Time: 25 Minutes

Cook Time: 55 Minutes

Servings: 5

Ingredients

- 2 Tbsp olive oil
- 1 lb small red potatoes, cut into thin slices
- 1 1/2 cups sliced cremini mushrooms
- 1/2 cup chopped fresh banana peppers
- 1/2 cup chopped onions
- 1 tsp Italian seasoning
- 8 oz precooked Italian-style chicken sausage, quartered lengthwise and cut into 1/4-inch slices
- 2 cups thinly sliced kale
- 1/4 cup grated Asiago cheese
- Nonstick cooking spray
- 4 eggs
- Salt and black pepper to taste

Instructions

1. In a large skillet, heat oil over medium heat. Add potatoes; cover and cook for 10 minutes, stirring once, until potatoes are nearly tender.

2. Add mushrooms, banana peppers, onion, and Italian seasoning; cook 3 minutes. Add sausage and kale; cook for 3 to 5 minutes, or until kale has wilted and all vegetables are tender. Sprinkle with cheese.

3. Meanwhile, spray a nonstick skillet with cooking spray. Heat over medium heat. Break eggs into skillet. Reduce heat to low; cook eggs for 3 to 4 minutes, or until whites are completely set and yolks start to thicken.

4. Serve fried eggs over hash. Season with salt and pepper.

Prep Time: 25 Minutes

Cook Time: 60 Minutes

Servings: 2

Ingredients

For the Sausage:

- 3/4 tsp dried sage, crushed
- 1/2 tsp kosher salt
- 1/2 tsp freshly ground black pepper
- 1/2 tsp dried thyme, crushed
- 1/2 tsp garlic powder
- 1/2 tsp onion powder
- 1/8 tsp cayenne
- 3/4 tsp fennel seeds
- 3/4 ground pork

For the Eggs and Greens:

- 1 Tbsp extra-virgin olive oil
- 1 bunch kale, stemmed, leaves coarsely chopped
- 1/4 cup no-sugar-added chicken broth
- 2 cloves garlic, peeled and thinly sliced

- Salt and black pepper
- 2 Tbsp ghee
- 4 eggs

Instructions

1. Preheat oven to 200°F.
2. For the sausage: In a medium bowl, combine sage, salt, pepper, thyme, garlic powder, onion powder, cayenne, and fennel seeds; mix well. Add pork and gently work with your hands until spices are evenly distributed in the meat. Shape into four 1/2-inch-thick patties.
3. Heat a large skillet over medium heat. Add patties; cook 8 minutes or until done (160°F), turning once. Transfer to a baking sheet and keep warm in the oven.
4. For the eggs and greens: Add olive oil to the pan. Turn heat to medium-high. Add garlic and cook until soft. Add kale, turn heat to high, and add broth. Cover and cook 4 to 5 minutes or until kale is wilted but still bright green. Uncover and cook, stirring occasionally, until all of the liquid has evaporated, another 1 to 2 minutes. Season to taste with salt and pepper.

Transfer to a bowl. Cover loosely with foil to keep warm.

5. If there is any liquid left in the skillet, wipe it out with a paper towel. Add ghee. When ghee is hot, gently break the eggs into the skillet. Turn heat to medium. Season with salt and pepper to taste. Cover and cook until whites are set and the edges are starting to turn crispy and brown.

6. To serve, top each sausage patty with a fried egg and serve with sautéed kale.

Prep Time: 15 Minutes

Cook Time: 50 Minutes

Servings: 4

Ingredients

- 1 can (14–16oz) black beans, drained
- Juice of 1 lime
- 1/4 tsp cumin
- Hot sauce
- 8 eggs
- Salt and black pepper to taste
- 1/2 cup feta cheese, plus more for serving
- Pico de Gallo or bottled salsa
- Sliced avocado (optional)

Instructions

1. Pulse the black beans, lime juice, cumin, and a few shakes of hot sauce in a food processor until it has the consistency of refried beans, adding a bit of water to help if necessary.

2. Coat a small nonstick pan with nonstick cooking spray or a bit of butter or olive oil and heat over medium heat.

3. Crack two eggs into a bowl and beat with a bit of salt and pepper.

4. Add the eggs to the pan, then use a spatula to stir and then lift the cooked egg on the bottom to allow raw egg to slide under.

5. When the eggs have all but set, spoon a quarter of the black bean mixture and 2 tablespoons feta down the middle of the omelet.

6. Use the spatula to fold over a third of the egg to cover the mixture in the center, then carefully slide the omelet onto a plate, using the spatula flip it over at the last second to form one fully rolled omelet.

7. Repeat with the remaining ingredients to make four omelets. Garnish with pico de gallo, avocado slices if you like, and bit more crumbled feta.

Prep Time: 15 Minutes

Cook Time: 50 Minutes

Servings: 4

Ingredients

- 1 can (16 oz) whole peeled tomatoes, with juice
- 1/2 small onion, chopped
- 1 clove garlic, chopped
- 1 Tbsp chopped chipotle pepper
- 1/4 cup chopped fresh cilantro
- Juice of 1 lime
- Salt and black pepper to taste
- 1 can (16 oz) black beans
- Pinch of ground cumin
- 8 eggs
- 8 corn tortillas

Instructions

1. Combine the tomatoes, onion, garlic, chipotle, cilantro, and half of the lime juice in a food processor

and pulse until well blended but still slightly chunky. Season with salt and pepper.

2. Mix the black beans, cumin, and remaining lime juice in a bowl; season with salt and pepper. Use the back of a fork to lightly mash up the beans, adding a splash of warm water if necessary.

3. Coat a large non-stick skillet or sauté pan with non-stick cooking spray and heat over medium heat. Break the eggs into the skillet; cook until the whites have set, but the yolks are still loose and runny.

4. On a separate burner, heat a medium skillet over medium heat and add the tortillas, 2 at a time; cook for 1 minute on each side, until lightly toasted.

5. To assemble the dish, spread the tortillas with the beans, top with the eggs, and top the eggs with the salsa. Garnish with more cilantro, if you like, and serve immediately.

Prep Time: 20 Minutes

Cook Time: 30 Minutes

Servings: 4-6

Ingredients

- 1 lb fresh brussels sprouts, ends trimmed and any yellowed/browned outer leaves removed, then sliced in half
- 3 Tbsp. olive oil, divided
- 1/2 tsp. Kosher salt
- 1/2 tsp. freshly-ground black pepper
- 1 lb (16 oz.) orecchiette (or any pasta)
- 4 chicken sausage links (I used spicy Italian), sliced into 1/4" thick coins
- 5 cloves garlic, peeled and thinly sliced
- 1/3 cup pesto
- Parmesan cheese, for serving

Instructions

1. Preheat oven to 400 degrees F. In a large bowl, mix together brussels sprouts, 2 Tbsp. olive oil, salt and pepper. Gently stir until well-combined.

2. Prepare a baking sheet with aluminum foil, then spread the brussels sprouts on it evenly. Roast for about 20-30 minutes, stirring once partway through, or until they are crispy on the outside and cooked on the inside. (My batch of tiny sprouts only took about 12 minutes to cook.) Remove from oven and set aside.

3. Meanwhile, heat the remaining olive oil in a skillet over medium-high heat. Add the sausage and cook, turning occasionally, until nearly-browned, about 6-8 minutes. Add the garlic, and continue cooking for another 1-2 minutes until the garlic is fragrant and the sausage is browned.

4. Cook the pasta in boiling water until al dente according to the package directions. (I begin heating my water while preparing the brussel sprouts, and added the pasta to the boiling water just after beginning to cook the sausage.) Once the pasta is cooked, drain the water (reserving 1/4 cup pasta water), and then toss together the pasta, pesto, cooked sausage and garlic, and brussels sprouts. Add in some

of the reserved pasta water if needed for extra moisture.

5. Serve warm, and sprinkle with freshly-grated Parmesan cheese.

10. Roasted Butternut Squash and Blackberry Harvest Salad

Prep Time: 20 Minutes

Cook Time: 30 Minutes

Servings: 6

Ingredients

Kale

- 10 oz. kale deboned and chopped
- 2-3 tablespoons olive oil
- 1/2 teaspoon salt
- Roasted Butternut Squash
- 1/2 butternut squash 24 ounces, cubed
- 1.5 tablespoons olive oil
- salt to taste
- pepper to taste
- Candied Nuts and Seeds
- 1 cup raw pecans
- 1/3 cup raw pumpkin seeds
- 1.5 tablespoons maple syrup
- 1/8 teaspoon sea salt

Balsamic Dressing:

- 1 teaspoon dijon mustard

- 1 tablespoon maple syrup

- 2 tablespoons balsamic vinegar

- 2 tablespoons olive oil

- 1/8 sea salt

Other Salad Ingredients

- 12 oz. blackberries

- 1/4 cup goat cheese

- 1/4 cup dried cranberries

Instructions

For the Kale

1. Place all ingredients for the kale in a large mixing bowl. Massage oil and salt into the kale with your hands for 3-4 minutes. Set aside.
2. For the Roasted Butternut Squash
3. Preheat the oven to 400°F and spray a baking sheet with olive oil cooking spray.
4. Spread butternut squash out on the baking sheet. Add olive oil, salt, and pepper to the butternut squash and toss until squash is evenly coated.

5. Place the baking sheet into the oven for 20-25 minutes.

For the Candied Nuts and Seeds

1. Prepare a baking sheet by spraying with olive oil cooking spray.
2. Place all ingredients for nuts into a medium mixing bowl. Toss until nuts are evenly coated and then spread out evenly onto the baking sheet.
3. Roast for 8-10 minutes at 400°F. You can roast the nuts in the oven with the squash.

For the Balsamic Dressing

1. Add all of the ingredients for the dressing into a mason jar. Tightly cover the mason jar and shake the jar to combine ingredients.

For the Salad

1. Add blackberries, goat cheese, cranberries, kale, nuts, and butternut squash into a large salad bowl. Pour dressing over the salad. Toss and enjoy!

11. Stovetop Southwest Tuna Mac and Cheese

Prep Time: 10 Minutes

Cook Time: 25 Minutes

Servings: 6

Ingredients

- 8 oz elbow noodles (or whatever noodles you'd like)
- 2 tablespoons butter
- 1 clove garlic, minced
- 1/4 cup whole wheat pastry flour (or sub regular flour or GF all purpose flour)
- ½ teaspoon onion powder
- 1 1/2 cups unsweetened cashew or almond milk
- Salt and pepper, to taste
- 6 oz sharp cheddar cheese (about 1 1/2 cups shredded cheddar cheese)
- 1 (1.1 ounce) packet taco seasoning (preferably organic)
- 1 (15 ounce) can black beans, rinsed and drained
- 1 (5 ounce) can yellowfin or albacore tuna, drained

- 2 oz sharp cheddar cheese, shredded and reserved for the topping (or about ½ cup shredded cheddar cheese)

To garnish:

- Chopped fresh cilantro
- Hot sauce, if desired

Instructions

2. First boil the noodles until al dente, according to the directions on the package. Once done cooking, drain and set aside.

3. While the noodles are boiling, make a slurry: In a large oven safe skillet or pot add butter and garlic. Once butter is melted, whisk in the flour and onion powder and cook for 30 seconds until a paste forms. Slowly add in cashew milk, whisking away any lumps.

4. Increase heat and bring mixture to a boil, then reduce heat and simmer for 5-10 minutes stirring every so often, until the sauce thickens up similar to a gravy

5. Next add in 6 oz cheese and 1 packet of taco seasoning and stir until completely melted.

6. Finally fold in cooked noodles, black beans and drained tuna and mix until well combined.

7. Top with 2 ounces of shredded cheddar. At this point you can either serve the mac and cheese and just fold in the extra cheddar you just added, or remove from heat and place under the broiler for 1-2 minutes or until cheese is bubbly and slightly golden. Serves 6. Top with cilantro and hot sauce if desired!

Prep Time: 20 Minutes

Cook Time: 15 Minutes

Servings: 4

Ingredients

- 1 ½ cups panko breadcrumbs
- Nonstick olive oil cooking spray
- 1 teaspoon salt
- 1 teaspoon black pepper
- 1 teaspoon onion powder
- 1 teaspoon paprika
- ½ teaspoon garlic powder
- 1/4 teaspoon cayenne pepper
- 2 large eggs
- 2 tablespoons almond milk (or milk of choice)
- 1 pound boneless skinless chicken breast, cut into into 1 inch cubes

Instructions

1. Preheat oven to 400 degrees F.

2. Add panko breadcrumbs to a large baking sheet and spread out in an even layer. Spray breadcrumbs with nonstick olive oil cooking spray. Bake for 2 minutes, then stir breadcrumbs (or just give the pan a shake) and then bake for 2-3 minutes or until breadcrumbs are golden brown. Keep heat in the oven.

3. Transfer breadcrumbs to a medium bowl. Whisk in spices: salt, black pepper, onion powder, paprika, garlic powder and cayenne pepper. Set aside.

4. In a separate medium bowl, whisk together the eggs and almond milk. Set aside.

5. Line the large baking sheet with an oven safe wire metal rack. Spray with nonstick cooking spray.

6. Dip each chicken cube into the egg mixture, then use a tong to grab each chicken nugget and toss into the breadcrumb mixture to completely coat with breadcrumbs. Use tongs to transfer to the wire rack, placing about 1 inch apart.

7. Generously spray the tops of the chicken nuggets with nonstick spray. Bake in the oven for 15-20 minutes until cooked through and temp reaches 165 degrees F with a meat thermometer. Serves 4. Serve with BBQ sauce, honey mustard, ketchup or whatever sauce you'd like!

Prep Time: 10 Minutes

Cook Time: 30 Minutes

Servings: 6

Ingredients

- 10 ounces dry pasta shells (or use rotini, fusilli, or whatever pasta you'd like)
- 3 tablespoons butter, divided
- 1 white onion, diced
- 8 ounces baby bella mushrooms, sliced
- 1 teaspoon dried thyme
- Salt and pepper, to taste
- 1/4 cup all purpose flour (or whole wheat flour or all purpose gluten free flour)
- 1 3/4 cup unsweetened almond milk (or cashew milk or regular milk)
- ½ teaspoon garlic powder
- 1/2 cup grated parmesan cheese
- 2 (5 ounce) cans tuna, drained
- 1 cup frozen peas
- Salt and pepper, to taste

For the topping:

- 1/2 cup breadcrumbs, gluten free if desired
- 1 tablespoon butter

Instructions

1. Preheat your oven to 350 degrees Spray a 2-quart baking dish or 9x9 inch baking pan with nonstick cooking spray, or grease with olive oil or butter.
2. First boil the noodles until al dente, according to the directions on the package. Once done cooking, drain and set aside.
3. Cook your mushrooms: Place a large pot over medium-high heat and add in 1 tablespoon butter. Once butter melts, add in the mushrooms, onions, thyme and salt and pepper. Stir occasionally until mushrooms and onions are cooked down about 4-6 minutes. Transfer to a bowl.
4. In the same skillet you cooked mushrooms, add in 2 tablespoons of butter and place over medium heat. Once butter is melted, whisk in a little bit of the flour and then slowly add in milk, a little bit at a time, alternating with the flour and vigorously whisking away any lumps. Bring mixture to a boil, then reduce

heat and simmer for a few minutes stirring every so often, until the sauce thickens up. If it gets too thick, add in ¼ cup more milk.

5. Once thick, turn off the heat and stir in garlic powder, parmesan cheese. salt and LOTS of freshly ground black pepper.

6. Stir in cooked noodles, mushroom and onion mixture, drained tuna and peas. Season again with salt and pepper, to taste. Pour mixture into your prepared baking pan.

7. In a small bowl, mix breadcrumbs with melted butter. Sprinkle breadcrumb mixture on top of casserole and bake for 20-30 minutes. Serves 6.

Prep Time: 40 Minutes

Cook Time: 20 Minutes

Servings: 4

Ingredients

- 1 pound boneless skinless chicken breast
- 1/4 cup low sodium soy sauce or coconut aminos
- 2 cloves garlic, minced
- 2 tablespoons brown sugar or coconut sugar
- 1 tablespoon tahini
- 1 tablespoon sesame oil (preferably toasted sesame oil)
- 1 tablespoon rice vinegar
- 1 tablespoon fresh grated ginger
- 1 tablespoon sesame seeds
- ½ teaspoon red pepper flakes

To garnish:

- Sliced green onion
- Sesame seeds

Instructions

1. In a large bowl, whisk together the soy sauce, garlic, brown sugar, tahini, sesame oil, rice vinegar, ginger, sesame seeds and red pepper flakes. Add chicken, then cover and place in the fridge for roughly 30 minutes or up to 24 hours. Then bake or grill your chicken however you like. Garnish with sliced green onion and additional sesame seeds.

2. To grill: Preheat the grill to 400 degrees F. Grill chicken for about 6-8 minutes per side; chicken is done when a meat thermometer reads 165 degrees F. Time will vary depending on the size of your chicken breast. Get all of my tips for grilling chicken.

3. If you'd like to bake the chicken, follow the instructions in this guide.

Prep Time: 15 Minutes

Cook Time: 40 Minutes

Servings: 6

Ingredients

For the chicken:

- 1 tablespoon olive oil
- 1 pound boneless skinless chicken thighs, diced into bite sized pieces
- Freshly ground salt and pepper

For the corn chowder:

- 1 medium white onion, chopped
- 3 garlic cloves, minced
- 1 poblano pepper, seeded and diced (can also use 1 seeded jalapeno)
- 1 red bell pepper, diced
- 4 cups diced yukon gold potatoes
- 5 cups fresh sweet corn off the cob (can also use frozen)
- 1 teaspoons cumin

- 1 teaspoon ground coriander
- 1/2 teaspoon ground turmeric
- ½ teaspoon chili powder
- 1/2 teaspoon garlic powder
- 1/2 teaspoon oregano
- Optional: ¼ teaspoon cayenne (only if you like a little heat)
- 2 cups milk of choice (I used unsweetened almond milk, but dairy milk or coconut milk would also work)
- 2 cups low sodium chicken broth
- ⅓ cup plain greek yogurt (or sour cream)
- 1 teaspoon salt, plus more to taste
- Freshly ground black pepper
- 1 (15 ounce) can black beans, rinsed and drained
- Juice from ½ lime

To garnish:

- Shredded sharp cheddar cheese
- Scallions
- 1/2 cup fresh diced cilantro
- Diced avocado
- Tortilla chips

1. In a large soup pot over medium-high heat add the olive oil and diced chicken, season with salt and pepper and cook until cooked through until chicken is no longer pink, about 5-7 minutes. Once chicken is done cooking, transfer to a bowl or plate and set aside.

2. In the same pot, reduce heat to medium and add in onion, garlic, poblano, red bell pepper, potatoes and corn and saute for 6-8 minutes or until potatoes start to soften a bit.

3. Next stir in spices and cook for 30 seconds to release their flavors and aromas, then slowly stir in the milk, broth and yogurt (or sour cream), scraping up any bits from the bottom of the pan as you stir. Season with salt and pepper. Reduce the heat to medium low and gently simmer for 10-15 minutes uncovered or until the potatoes are tender and can easily be pierced with a fork.

4. To give a creamy texture, blend approximately half of the soup (BE CAREFUL WHILE DOING THIS!) then return to the pot. Stir to incorporate and then taste and adjust seasonings -- adding in more salt and pepper if necessary. You can blend more if you like a

creamier soup, but I love a little texture. Finally stir in the chicken, black beans and lime juice.

5. To serve, garnish with shredded cheese, scallions, cilantro, avocado and a swirl of sour cream (if not vegan). Makes 6 servings.

Prep Time: 45 Minutes

Cook Time: 15 Minutes

Servings: 4

Ingredients

For the chicken:

- Grilled Sesame Chicken

For the salad:

- 4 cups shredded green cabbage
- 2 cups shredded red cabbage
- 1/2 cup diced green onion
- 3/4 cup freshly diced cilantro
- 1 cup shredded carrots (bagged or cut into matchsticks for excellent crunch!)
- 1 red bell pepper, thinly julienned
- 1 jalapeno, seeded and diced

For the dressing:

- 1 batch Sesame Ginger Dressing

For serving:

- 1/3 cup toasted sliced almonds
- 1/3 cup roasted cashews halves
- Sesame seeds
- Extra cilantro
- Extra green onion
- A few jalapeno slices
- Optional: Crispy wonton strips

Instructions

1. Marinate the chicken using this grilled sesame chicken.
2. Make the sesame ginger dressing. Set aside.
3. Assemble the salad together: in a large bowl, add the green and red cabbage, green onion, cilantro, carrots, bell pepper and jalapeno. Pour dressing all over the salad and toss to combine and coat all the veggies. Cover and set aside while you bake or grill your chicken according to the recipe.
4. Serve the salad: add salad to a large platter. Garnish with toasted sliced almonds, cashews, extra cilantro, a sprinkle of sesame seeds, a few jalapeno slices and some additional chopped green onion, if desired. I also love adding crispy wonton strips but that's totally

optional. Dig in! Serves 4 as a hearty main dish or 6 as a side dish.

Prep Time: 15 Minutes

Cook Time: 30 Minutes

Servings: 4

Ingredients

For the brown butter:

- 1/4 cup salted butter
- For the corn:
- 1 tablespoon butter or olive oil
- 3 cups fresh sweet corn, cut off the cob (3-4 ears of corn should yield roughly 3 cups)
- Freshly ground salt and pepper, to taste

For the ricotta:

- 1/2 cup ricotta
- ½ teaspoon salt
- For the pasta:
- 10 oz tagliatelle pasta (or sub fettuccine or linguine or any type of pasta you want!)
- 3/4 cup reserved pasta water

To garnish:

- 1/4 cup basil, cut into ribbons
- 1/4 cup sliced green onions

Instructions

1. First, brown your butter: add butter to a medium saucepan or skillet and place over medium heat. The butter will begin to melt, crackle, and then eventually foam. Make sure you whisk constantly during this process. After a couple of minutes, the butter will begin to brown and turn a nice golden amber color on the bottom of the saucepan, this usually happens once it foams. Continue to whisk and remove from heat as soon as the butter begins to brown and give off a nutty aroma. Immediately transfer the butter to a medium bowl to prevent burning, making sure you scrape all the yummy brown bits from the pan with a rubber spatula; this is where the flavor is! Set aside to cool.

2. Bring a large pot of water to a boil for your pasta, then start cooking your corn.

3. Place a skillet over medium high heat and add in 1 tablespoon olive oil or butter. Once oil is hot or butter is melted, add in the corn, season with salt and

pepper, and saute for approximately 10 minutes; stirring every so often until corn begins to caramelize and turn slightly golden in places. Add half of the sauteed corn to a blender with the ½ cup of ricotta and ½ teaspoon salt and set aside; do not blend yet. Reserve the remaining half of corn for stirring into the pasta.

4. While the corn is cooking, you can cook your pasta according to the directions on the package. Before draining pasta and adding back to the pan, reserve ½ cup of pasta water and add to the corn/ricotta mixture, then blend the mixture until mostly smooth.

5. Finally, add brown butter to the cooked pasta and stir to coat, then toss in the blended corn/ricotta mixture, extra corn, basil and green onion. Add freshly ground salt and pepper to taste. If you like a little heat, i think red pepper flakes would be fabulous. Serves 4-6.

Prep Time: 25 Minutes

Cook Time: 30 Minutes

Servings: 4

Ingredients

For the zucchini boats:

- Olive oil
- 4 medium zucchini, sliced in half lengthwise (look for zucchini that is similar in size)
- Freshly ground salt and pepper

For the buffalo mac and cheese:

- 8 ounces dry elbow noodles
- 2 tablespoons salted butter
- ¼ cup all purpose flour (or sub whole wheat or GF all purpose flour)
- 1/2 teaspoon garlic powder
- 1/4 teaspoon onion powder
- 1 3/4 cups unsweetened cashew milk, almond milk or regular milk

- 6 oz sharp cheddar cheese (about 1 ½ heaping cup shredded sharp cheddar cheese off the block)
- Freshly ground salt and pepper, to taste
- 1/2 cup medium to hot buffalo sauce

For topping:

- 1/2 cup shredded cheddar cheese
- 1/2 cup panko breadcrumbs
- 1 tablespoon melted butter

For garnish:

- Sliced green onion

Instructions

1. Preheat the oven to 400 degrees. Grease a 9x13 inch pan with olive oil or line a large baking sheet with parchment paper.
2. Using a spoon, scoop centers from zucchini while leaving a 1/4-inch rim to create boats. Place zucchini in the greased pan; they should snuggle pretty tightly in there, but if you can't fit them all in, you can use two pans. Brush zucchini with a little olive oil (about 1 tablespoon or so). You can also simply spray them

with an all natural oil-only cooking spray. Generously season with salt and pepper.

3. Boil the noodles in a large pot until al dente, according to the directions on the package. Once done cooking, drain and return noodles to the large pot.

4. While the noodles are boiling, make your mac and cheese sauce: in a medium pot or skillet, add butter and place over medium heat. Once butter is melted, whisk in a little bit of the flour and then slowly add in milk, a little bit at a time, alternating with the flour and vigorously whisking away any lumps. Bring mixture to a boil, then reduce heat and simmer for a few minutes stirring every so often, until the sauce thickens up a bit. Stir in garlic powder, onion powder, salt and LOTS of freshly ground black pepper.

5. Next add in 1 cup of shredded sharp cheddar cheese to the sauce and stir until completely melted. Pour the cheese sauce over the noodles, then add in buffalo sauce. Stir to completely coat the noodles.

6. Spoon mac and cheese evenly into zucchini boats. Cover with foil, and bake for 20 minutes or until zucchini is slightly fork tender.

7. Remove from oven and top each with 1 tablespoon of shredded cheddar cheese. In a small bowl, mix

breadcrumbs with melted butter. Sprinkle breadcrumb mixture on top of zucchini boats. Bake for 5-10 more minutes until breadcrumbs become slightly golden. Garnish with green onion before serving and drizzle with some ranch or bleu cheese dressing, if desired. Serves 4; 2 boats per person.

Prep Time: 20 Minutes

Cook Time: 10 Minutes

Servings: 6

Ingredients

Cobb Chicken Salad:

- 1 medium rotisserie chicken deboned and shredded
- 4 hard-boiled eggs diced
- 4 strips thick-cut cooked bacon chopped
- 1 cup cherry tomatoes halved
- 1/3 cup red onion finely diced
- 1 cup yellow corn
- salt and pepper to taste
- 6-8 cups chopped romaine

Greek Yogurt Blue Cheese Dressing

- 1/2 cup plain Greek yogurt any fat percentage works
- 2 oz. blue cheese crumbles
- 1/2 teaspoon apple cider vinegar
- 1 tablespoon lemon juice
- 1 tablespoon water

- 1/8 teaspoon black pepper

- 1/8 teaspoon salt or to taste

Instructions

Greek Yogurt Blue Cheese Dressing

1. First, prepare the Greek Yogurt Blue Cheese Dressing.
2. Place all ingredients for the dressing into a small bowl and mix.
3. Use a fork to partially break up the blue cheese into smaller chunks.
4. Add more water as needed to thin out the dressing to your desire.
5. Set aside for later.

Cobb Chicken Salad

1. First, debone and shred a medium rotisserie chicken. Set aside.
2. Next, prepare hard-boiled eggs. Bring a medium-pot of water to a rolling boil over high heat. Then, add eggs to the water. Continue boiling for 8 minutes. Remove from water immediately and transfer to an ice bath for 5 minutes before peeling and chopping. Set aside.

3. Prepare veggies by halving cherry tomatoes and finely dicing red onion.

4. Prepare bacon by pan-frying 4 strips of thick-cut bacon over medium/high heat for around 10 minutes or until your bacon has reached the desired texture. Remove excess grease with a paper towel and then roughly chop.

5. Finally, assemble salad. Place shredded chicken, hard-boiled eggs, bacon, cherry tomatoes, red onion, and yellow corn into a large bowl. Toss until combined.

6. Pour in Greek yogurt dressing and toss one more time. Season with salt and pepper, to taste.

7. Serve immediately tossed with 1-2 cups of romaine lettuce or meal-prep for later by keeping the chicken salad and romaine separate.

Prep Time: 30 Minutes

Cook Time: 25 Minutes

Servings: 16

Ingredients

Veggies:

- 5 bell peppers any color, thinly sliced
- 1 large yellow onion thinly sliced
- 2 tablespoons olive oil
- 2 tablespoons taco seasoning
- Rice
- 1 cup long-grain white rice
- 2.25 cups water

Beef:

- 2 lbs. 85% ground beef
- 2 tablespoons tomato paste
- 5 tablespoons taco seasoning
- ¾ cup water
- Other
- 8 oz. shredded white cheddar cheese

- 16 large flour tortillas

Instructions

Veggies

- First, preheat oven to 375°F.
- Then, prepare bell peppers and onion by thinly slicing.
- Place veggies on a large baking sheet and drizzle with olive oil.
- Then, season with taco seasoning and toss.
- Bake at 375°F for 20-25 minutes or until onions become translucent.
- Set aside.

Rice

1. Place 1 cup of white rice and 2.25 cups of water into a small bot.
2. Bring to a boil over medium/high heat.
3. Once boiling, reduce heat to low and cover. Let simmer for around 15-20 minutes or until all water absorbs.

Beef

1. While the veggies are cooking, heat a large nonstick skillet over medium/high heat.
2. Then, add in ground beef and saute for 7-10 minutes or until almost fully browned.
3. Add in tomato paste, taco seasoning, and water and continue cooking for a few more minutes until liquid reduces.
4. Set aside.

Beef Burritos

1. Prepare beef burritos by laying out all 16 flour tortillas.
2. Then, evenly distribute beef, veggies, and rice.
3. Finally, sprinkle on a handful of cheese.
4. Tightly wrap each burrito by folding the sides in and rolling.
5. Then, wrap each individual burrito in a piece of tin foil and remove as much air as possible.
6. Store in the freezer for up to 3 months.

21. Cilantro Lime Shrimp Bowls

Prep Time: 15 Minutes

Cook Time: 45 Minutes

Servings: 4

Ingredients

For the Brown Rice

- 1 cup short grain brown rice
- 2 cups water
- For the Slaw
- 2 cups shredded carrots
- 2 cups shredded purple cabbage
- 1/4 cup rice vinegar
- 2 tablespoons lime juice
- 1/8 teaspoon salt or more to taste
- 1 tablespoon maple syrup

For the Greek Yogurt Dressing

- 1/2 cup plain, nonfat Greek yogurt
- 1 tablespoon olive oil

- 1 teaspoon garlic powder

- 2 tablespoons lime juice

- pinch of salt

For the Cilantro Lime Shrimp

- 1 lb. pre-cooked shrimp tails-off

- 1 teaspoon coconut oil

- 1 tablespoon minced garlic

- 2 tablespoons lime juice

- salt and pepper to taste

- 2 tablespoons fresh chopped chopped cilantro

- 1 teaspoon cumin

Instructions

For the Brown Rice

1. Place 1 cup of short grain brown rice and 2 cups of water into a medium size pot. Turn to high and bring to a rolling boil. Cover and turn to low. Let simmer for around 30-35 minutes or until all of the liquid has absorbed.

For the Slaw

1. Place 2 cups of shredded carrots and 2 cups of shredded purple cabbage in a large bowl.
2. Prep dressing by mixing together rice vinegar, lime juice, salt, and maple syrup together. Then, pour over veggies.
3. Toss.

Greek Yogurt Dressing

1. Whisk together Greek yogurt, olive oil, garlic powder, and lime juice.

Cilantro Lime Shrimp

1. Place coconut oil and garlic in a large sauce pan. Heat to medium/high heat. Add in shrimp and sautee for 2-3 minutes, just enough to heat them up.
2. Squeeze on lime juice, season with salt and pepper, cumin, and fresh cilantro.
3. Note: There will be a sauce of sorts that is created from the shrimp. We recommend pouring it over the rice!

For Serving

1. Serve with a handful of arugula.

Prep Time: 20 Minutes

Cook Time: 25 Minutes

Servings: 4

Ingredients

- 1 lb. cooked shredded chicken breast
- 6 slices of bacon chopped
- 1 cup cherry tomatoes halved
- 1/4 cup red onion finely diced
- 1 cup chopped kale deboned
- 1 teaspoon olive oil
- 1/2 cup plain Greek yogurt
- 1 teaspoon ranch seasoning
- 1/2 tablespoon lemon juice
- 1/2 teaspoon vinegar-based hot sauce or more, to taste

Instructions

2. First, make your massaged kale. Place kale into a medium bowl and drizzle on a teaspoon of olive oil.

Then, use your hands to massage the oil into the kale for 3-5 minutes or until the kale becomes wilted and broken down.

3. Place shredded chicken, bacon, cherry tomatoes, red onion, and massaged kale into a large bowl. Mix and set aside.

4. Create the sauce by mixing together plain Greek yogurt, ranch seasoning, lemon juice, and hot sauce.

5. Add sauce to the shredded chicken mixture and mix until combined.

Prep Time: 30 Minutes

Cook Time: 25 Minutes

Servings: 4

Ingredients

Pesto Chicken:

- 16 oz. boneless skinless chicken breasts
- 1/3 cup pesto (we used homemade)
- Roasted Asparagus
- 1 lb. asparagus
- 1/2 tablespoon olive oil
- salt and pepper, to taste

Quinoa:

- 1 cup quinoa, uncooked
- 2 cups water
- Mozzarella and Tomato Salad
- 1/2 cup mozzarella pearls
- 10 oz. cherry tomatoes, halved
- 1/2 tablespoon olive oil
- 1/2 tablespoon balsamic vinegar

- 1/4 medium red onion, very thinly sliced
- salt and pepper, to taste

Optional toppings

- 1/4 cup toasted pine nuts
- 1/2 cup pesto
- 1/4 cup grated parmesan cheese

Instructions

Pesto Chicken

1. First, preheat oven to 375°F and spray a baking sheet with nonstick cooking spray.
2. Prep chicken by placing chicken breast into a gallon-size bag and pouring on pesto. Close bag and give your chicken a good shake, making sure it's covered in pesto. Place in the refrigerator for 30 minutes to marinate (option to do this the night before and let sit for 12-24 hours).
3. Once marinated, transfer chicken breast to baking sheet. Make sure you put all that excess pesto on top of the chicken breast. Bake at 375°F for about 20-25 minutes depending on the size of your breasts.
4. Remove from oven, let cool, and slice into cubes.

Roasted Asparagus

1. Prepare asparagus by placing spears on a baking sheet. Drizzle with olive oil and season with salt and pepper.
2. Bake at 375°F for about 10-12 minutes. Make sure you don't overcook your asparagus, no one likes mushy spears!

Quinoa

1. Place quinoa and water into a medium pot. Bring to a boil. Then, cover and turn heat down to low. Let simmer for about 20 minutes or until all liquid has absorbed.
2. Mozzarella and Tomato Salad
3. Begin by slicing cherry tomatoes in half. Place them into a medium-size bowl.
4. Add in mozzarella pearls, olive oil, balsamic vinegar, sliced onion, salt, and pepper.
5. Mix and set aside.
6. Bowl Assembly
7. This recipe serves 4, so separate everything out into 4 portions.

8. Serve with more fresh pesto on top of the chicken, toasted pine nuts on top of the asparagus, and a sprinkle of parmesan on top of the entire thing.

Prep Time: 20 Minutes

Cook Time: 15 Minutes

Servings: 8

Ingredients

- 2 tablespoons olive oil
- 1 lb. ground beef any kind of ground meat will work
- 1 medium onion diced
- 1 tablespoon minced garlic
- 2 tablespoons chili powder
- 1/2 teaspoon smoked paprika
- 1 teaspoon ground cumin
- 1/2 teaspoon red pepper flakes
- 1/4 teaspoon pepper
- 1/4 teaspoon salt
- 2 tablespoons hot sauce
- 1 large red pepper diced
- 1 large green pepper diced
- 1 cup uncooked long grain white rice
- 5 cups beef broth divided
- 1 15-oz. can tomato sauce

- 1 15-oz. can diced tomatoes
- 1 4-oz. can green chiles

Instructions

1. Turn on the Instant Pot's saute function and add olive oil.
2. When olive oil is fragrant, add onion and garlic. Cook for one minute and then add ground beef.
3. Saute beef for 3-4 minutes, partially browning.
4. Turn saute function off and add the rest of the ingredients (only 4 cups of broth) to the Instant Pot and stir until all ingredients are combined.
5. Cover Instant Pot, seal valve, and cook for 3 minutes on high pressure.
6. When your Instant Pot beeps, quick release and let out the steam. Then, open Instant Pot.
7. Add the last cup of broth (or more if desired) and stir.
8. Serve stuffed pepper soup with Greek yogurt and green onions.

Prep Time: 20 Minutes

Cook Time: 20 Minutes

Servings: 4

Ingredients

For the carrots:

- 4 large carrots, cut in half vertically and stems/tops removed
- 1 tablespoon avocado oil
- Freshly ground salt and pepper

For the salad:

- 5 ounces baby arugula
- ¾ cup dried fig halves
- 1/3 cup walnuts halves and pieces
- 1/3 cup goat cheese crumbles
- 1 avocado, sliced

Maple Tahini Dressing:

- ¼ cup drippy tahini (I always use Soom Tahini)

- 2 tablespoons fresh lemon juice

- 1-2 teaspoons pure maple syrup

- ½ teaspoon dijon mustard

- ¼ teaspoon garlic powder

- 2-3 tablespoons warm water, to thin out a bit

- ¼ teaspoon salt

- Freshly ground black pepper

Instructions

1. Add vertically cut carrots to a large bowl or a platter and drizzle with avocado oil then season with freshly ground salt and pepper. Use tongs or clean hands to coat the carrots with the oil.

2. Preheat the grill to medium high heat (about 400 degrees F) and grill the carrots for 15-25 minutes total or until slightly tender, flipping halfway through. Please note, if you don't want to grill your carrots, you can roast them at 400 degrees F for 30 minutes or until tender on a baking sheet lined with parchment paper.

3. Toast walnuts in a dry skillet over medium heat, stirring occasionally until toasted and fragrant, about 5 minutes. Set aside.

4. While the carrots are cooking you can make your dressing: in a medium bowl, whisk together the tahini, lemon juice, maple syrup, dijon, garlic powder, water (1 tablespoon at a time until you reach your desired consistency) and salt and pepper. Set aside.

5. Add arugula to a large platter (or you can keep it in a large bowl) and then layer with the toppings: grilled carrots, dried fig halves, toasted walnuts, goat cheese crumbles and avocado slices.

6. Drizzle tahini dressing all over the top and season with freshly ground salt and pepper. Divide into bowls and enjoy! Salad keeps well for 2-4 days. Serves 4 as a main and 6 as a side salad.

Prep Time: 20 Minutes

Cook Time: 15 Minutes

Servings: 6

Ingredients

For the grilled corn:

- 4 ears of corn
- 1 tablespoon avocado oil
- Freshly ground salt and pepper

For the salad:

- 1 ½ cups halved cherry tomatoes (i love heirloom cherry or grape tomatoes!)
- 1 avocado, diced
- 1/3 cup goat cheese crumbled
- ¼ cup diced red onion or sub green onion
- 6 large leaves basil, julienned

Hot Honey Vinaigrette:

- 2 tablespoons avocado oil or olive oil

- 1 tablespoon honey
- Pinch of cayenne pepper OR 1/2 teaspoon hot sauce of choice
- 2 teaspoons apple cider vinegar (or sub fresh lime juice)
- ¼ teaspoon dijon mustard
- ⅛ teaspoon garlic powder
- Freshly ground salt and pepper, to taste

Instructions

1. Preheat grill to medium high heat.
2. Drizzle corn with oil and rub all over. Season with salt and pepper. Place the corn directly on the grill and turn occasionally until the corn is charred and cooked, about 20 minutes.
3. Allow corn to cool then cut the corn from the cob and place in a large bowl. Add tomatoes, avocado, goat cheese, red onion and basil. Toss together to combine.
4. Make your hot honey vinaigrette: in a mason jar or small bowl add honey and cayenne or hot sauce; microwave for 10-15 seconds until the honey is hot.

Remove and add in the olive oil, apple cider vinegar, dijon, garlic powder and salt and pepper; put a lid on the mason jar and shake well to combine. You can also whisk together in a small bowl if preferred. Taste and add more hot sauce or cayenne if you want it spicier! Pour over the corn salad and toss to combine. Season the salad with salt and pepper to taste.

5. Enjoy the corn salad immediately. If you are making ahead of time, I recommend leaving the avocado and goat cheese out until ready to serve.

Prep Time: 30 Minutes

Cook Time: 30 Minutes

Servings: 8

Ingredients

Kale Slaw

- 1 cup packed kale, de-boned, rinsed and chopped
- 1 teaspoon olive oil
- pinch of salt
- 2 tablespoons minced red onion
- 1 large radish, thinly sliced
- 1/2 teaspoon apple cider vinegar
- 1 teaspoon lime juice
- Sweet Potatoe Taco Meat
- 1 large sweet potato, chopped into 1-inch squares
- 2 cloves garlic, minced
- 1 tablespoon olive oil
- 1/2 tablespoon chili powder
- 1/2 tablespoon ground cumin
- 1/8 teaspoon paprika

- 1/2 teaspoon salt
- 1 15-oz. can garbanzo beans, (drained, rinsed, and de-cased)

Cilantro Lime Quinoa

- 1/2 cup uncooked quinoa
- 1 cup water
- 2 tablespoons fresh cilantro, finely chopped
- 1 teaspoon lime juice
- pinch of salt
- Tacos
- 8 small flour tortillas
- 1 large avocado
- salsa or hot sauce

Instructions

Kale Slaw

1. Place kale into a medium mixing bowl. Add olive oil and massage with your hands for 3-4 minutes or until kale breaks down and becomes soft.
2. Add the rest of the ingredients for the kale slaw to the bowl and mix. Make sure all ingredients are combined and place into the refrigerator.

Sweet Potato Taco Meat

1. First, preheat oven to 400°F. Place sweet potato and garlic onto a baking sheet. Drizzle with olive oil and then season with chili powder, cumin, paprika, salt, and pepper. Toss and make sure all ingredients are combined and sweet potatoes are covered with olive oil and spices. Roast for 10 minutes.
2. Remove from oven and add garbanzo beans to the baking sheet. Toss with all ingredients and roast for an additional 15 minutes.
3. Begin to prepare cilantro lime quinoa and then remove sweet potatoes from the oven.

Cilantro Lime Quinoa

1. Place water and quinoa into a medium saucepan over
    high heat. Bring to a boil and then turn heat to low,
    cover, and let simmer until all water has been
    absorbed (about 20 minutes).
2. Next, place quinoa into a mixing bowl and add
    cilantro, lime juice, and salt. Mix well.

Tacos

1. Evenly distribute kale, sweet potatoes, cilantro lime
    quinoa, and an avocado onto tortillas and enjoy with
    your favorite salsa or hot sauce.

Prep Time: 20 Minutes

Cook Time: 25 Minutes

Servings: 4

Ingredients

Tabouli

- 1 cup cooked quinoa (here's how to make it in the Instant Pot!)
- 1 cup fresh finely chopped parsley
- 1 cup finely chopped fresh arugula
- 1/4 cup red onion, finely diced
- 1/2 cup cherry tomatoes, diced
- Dressing
- 1 tablespoon balsamic vinegar
- 1 tablespoon apple cider vinegar
- 2 tablespoons olive oil
- 1 tablespoon lemon juice
- salt and pepper to taste

Instructions

1. Add all ingredients for the tabouli in a large mixing bowl. Set aside.

2. Then, add all dressing ingredients to a mason jar and cover. Shake dressing until on ingredients are combined.

3. Pour dressing over tabouli and mix well.

4. Serve and enjoy!

Prep Time: 20 Minutes

Cook Time: 25 Minutes

Servings: 6

Ingredients

Potato Salad

- 1/2 lb. cooked bacon chopped into bite-sized pieces
- 4 cups chopped Idaho potatoes 1.5-inch cubes (skin on)
- 2 hard-boiled eggs chopped
- 1/2 cup shredded cheddar cheese
- 2 tablespoons minced chives

Potato Salad Sauce

- 3/4 cup plain nonfat Greek yogurt
- 3 tablespoons avocado mayonnaise
- 2 teaspoon dijon mustard
- 3 teaspoons dill pickle juice
- 2 tablespoons minced dill pickles
- 1/8 teaspoon salt
- 1/8 teaspoon ground pepper

Instructions

1. Begin, by cooking bacon by following our Oven Bacon tutorial. Once cooked, remove any excess grease and then chop into bite-sized pieces. Set aside.

2. Next, bring a large pot of water to a boil and add potatoes to the pot. Boil until potatoes are cooked, but still firm.

3. While potatoes are boiling, mix all ingredients for the potato salad sauce in a medium bowl. Set aside.

4. When potatoes are done cooking, remove from heat and strain water.

5. Add potatoes to a large bowl along with the chopped bacon, hard boiled eggs, shredded cheddar cheese, and chives. Mix well.

6. Finally, pour potato salad sauce over the potato mixture and mix until sauce is covering all of the ingredients. Mash the potatoes with a wooden spoon (just a little bit) to create a creamy potato salad consistency.

7. Eat immediately or chill in the fridge to eat cold for later.

Prep Time: 20 Minutes

Cook Time: 2hrs 25 Minutes

Servings: 4

Ingredients

- 1 lb. cooked, shredded chicken breast
- 1 large green apple finely chopped
- 1/4 cup red onion finely diced
- 2 large celery stalks finely diced
- 1/3 cup dried cranberries or Craisins
- 1/2 cup nonfat Greek yogurt
- 1 tablespoon lemon juice
- 1 tablespoon honey
- 1/2 teaspoon garlic powder
- 1/8 teaspoon salt
- pepper to taste

Instructions

1. Place shredded chicken, green apple, red onion, celery, and dried cranberries into a large bowl. Mix and set aside.
2. Create the sauce by mixing together Greek yogurt, lemon juice, honey, garlic powder, salt, and pepper.
3. Add sauce to the shredded chicken mixture and mix until combined.